This notebook belongs to:

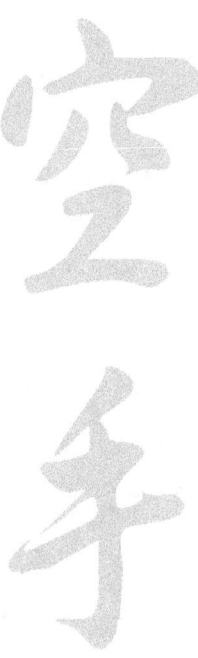

ISBN: 9781071398333
Independently published
martialnotebooks@gmail.com

Number	Character	*On* reading		General reading
1	一	ichi	いち	ichi
2	二	ni	に	ni
3	三	san	さん	san
4	四	shi	し	yon
5	五	go	ご	go
6	六	roku	ろく	roku
7	七	shichi	しち	nana
8	八	hachi	はち	hachi
9	九	ku, kyū	く, きゅう	kyū
10	十	jū	じゅう	jū
13	十三	jū-san	じゅうさん	jū-san
20	二十 / 廿	ni-jū	にじゅう	ni-jū
30	三十 / 卅	san-jū	さんじゅう	san-jū
40	四十	shi-jū	しじゅう	yon-jū
50	五十	go-jū	ごじゅう	go-jū
60	六十	roku-jū	ろくじゅう	roku-jū
70	七十	shichi-jū	しちじゅう	nana-jū
80	八十	hachi-jū	はちじゅう	hachi-jū
90	九十	ku-jū	くじゅう	kyū-jū
100	百	hyaku	ひゃく	hyaku
1,000	千	sen	せん	sen

Date

Date

Date

Date

Date

空手

Date

Date

Date

Date

Date

Date

空手

Date

Date

Date

Date

空手

Date

Date

空手

Date

Date

空手

Date

Date

空手

Date

Date

Date

Date

Date

Date

空手

Date

Date

Date

Date

Date

Date

空手

Date

Date

Date

Date

Date

Date

空手

Date

Date

空手

Date

Date

Date

Date

空手

Date

Date

Date

Date

空手

Date

Date

空手

Date

Date

Date

Date

Date

Date

空手

Date

Date

Date

Date

空手

Date

Date

空手

Date

Date

Date

Date

Date

Date

Date

Date

空手

Date

Date

Date

Date

Date

Date

Date

Date

空手

Date

Date

空手

Date

Date

空手

Date

Date

Date

Date

Date

Date

Date

Date

Date

Date

Date

Date

Date

Date

Date

www.ingramcontent.com/pod-product-compliance
Lightning Source LLC
Chambersburg PA
CBHW070433290526
45791CB00005B/1960